Simplified Solution Approach To **ANOREXIA NERVOSA**

Breaking Chains, Restoring Lives: Your Comprehensive Guide to Overcoming Anorexia Nervosa Through Empowerment and Resilience

Dr QUENTIN GLYN

Table Of Contents

CHAPTER ONE
Anorexia Nervosa

Extreme thinness brought on by self-imposed fasting and a distorted body image are hallmarks of anorexia nervosa, a complicated and dangerous mental health illness.

A thorough and straightforward solution method is essential while treating and managing anorexia nervosa.

Understanding the disease, addressing its incidence and demography, and emphasizing the value of support and intervention should all be part of this strategy.

Definition And Synopsis

As one of a range of eating disorders, anorexia nervosa is characterized by a continuous limitation of caloric intake, a strong fear of gaining weight or becoming obese, and a disruption of one's self-image. Anorexics often have a skewed impression of their size and weight, which causes them to engage in obsessive exercise, excessive diets, and other actions meant to stop weight gain.

Demographics And Prevalence

Although illness may afflict anyone of any age, gender, or background, teenagers and young adults are the most likely age group to get a diagnosis of anorexia nervosa. In

Western countries, where there is a greater focus on thinness and beauty standards, disordered eating patterns may arise and an increased risk of anorexia is shown. However, it's important to understand that anorexia nervosa affects people all over the world and that social and cultural aspects should be taken into account in treatment efforts.

Consequences For Mental And Physical Health

The effects of anorexia nervosa may be rather detrimental to one's physical and emotional well-being. Malnutrition, electrolyte imbalances, cardiac issues, and perhaps organ failure are among the physical consequences. An elevated risk of suicide as well as anxiety and sadness are all included in the mental health effects. It is essential to identify and treat anorexia as soon as possible in order to avoid these long-term health effects.

Economic And Social Burden

Anorexia Nervosa has a substantial negative impact on society and the economy in addition to personal health. The financial burden of medical care, therapy, and missed productivity is high. In addition, the illness may cause interpersonal conflicts and social isolation, which impacts the person's family and community in addition to themselves.

Dispelling Myths And Raising Awareness

In order to treat anorexia nervosa, it is necessary to dispel the stigma around eating disorders and mental health. Early diagnosis and intervention may be facilitated by fostering open communication and raising awareness. A setting that is accepting and supportive may encourage those who suffer from anorexia to seek assistance.

Methods Of Holistic Therapy

Applying comprehensive treatment methods is a straightforward solution approach to anorexia nervosa. A mix of dietary, psychological, and medicinal therapies are included in this. Given the complex nature of the condition, cooperation amongst medical professionals—such as doctors, therapists, and dietitians—is crucial.

Family And Support Systems Involved

In order to heal, family and social support are essential. Better communication and the creation of a supportive atmosphere are two benefits of including family in the treatment process. Teaching friends and relatives about anorexia nervosa may improve comprehension and dispel myths, leading to a more sympathetic attitude.

Education And Prevention Initiatives

The two main strategies for treating anorexia nervosa are education campaigns and prevention programs. Together, community groups, healthcare practitioners, and schools may launch awareness programs that educate people about nutrition, good body image, and the possible dangers of severe dieting.

In conclusion, a simple strategy for treating anorexia nervosa entails comprehending the condition, identifying the demographics and prevalence of the condition, and realizing the significance of support and intervention. In order to help those impacted by Anorexia Nervosa and lessen the effects of this major mental health disease, we may strive toward a more holistic approach that addresses the physical and mental health consequences, and social and economic costs, and promotes awareness and prevention.

CHAPTER TWO

Unpacking The Nervous System

1.   Defined Terms And Diagnostic Standards:

Anorexia Nervosa (AN) is a severe mental illness that is characterized by an extreme fear of gaining weight and a skewed perception of one's body, which causes self-imposed starvation and significant weight loss. Along with an intense need to be slim, people with AN often have an obsession with eating, diets, and body size.

Diagnostic Standards: The DSM-5 (Diagnostic and Statistical Manual of

Mental Disorders, Fifth Edition) lists the following as diagnostic standards:

Food restriction: People severely restrict their food intake, which results in a noticeably low body weight.

Extreme fear of gaining weight: Even if a person is underweight, they may have an unreasonable dread of gaining weight or becoming fat.

Warped body image: When someone has a distorted self-perception, they may believe they are overweight even when they are really underweight.

When women of reproductive age do not have at least three consecutive monthly cycles, it is known as amenorrhea (in females). This condition is sometimes brought on by significant weight loss.

2. Subtypes And Differences:

Subcategories:

Restricting Type: People mostly cut down on their food intake and practice severe fasting or dieting.

Type of Binge Eating/Purging: When someone has a binge-eating episode, they may compensate by overindulging in exercise or self-inflicted vomiting.

Changes:

Atypical Anorexia Nervosa: People who fit all the criteria for AN may not seem underweight because of things like muscle mass in athletes or growth spurts in teenagers.

Purging Disorder: Not as severe in weight loss as Anorexia Nervosa, but comparable to it.

3. Causes And Precursors

Etiology (Root Causes):

Biological Factors: Research indicates a greater risk if an eating problem exists or has been in a family member. Genetic predisposition also plays a part.

Psychological factors: worry, perfectionism, low self-esteem, and body dissatisfaction all play a part.

Sociocultural Factors: The development of AN is influenced by media influence, cultural standards of beauty, and societal demands to be slim.

Hazardous Elements

Gender: More common in women, yet it may also impact men.

Age: Can develop at any age, but usually starts in adolescence.

Occupation: Because of performance-related weight demands, athletes, dancers, and models may be more vulnerable.

Simplified Method of Solving:

Early Intervention:

Education: Spread knowledge of AN and its symptoms.

Screening: Make screenings a routine practice, particularly for high-risk populations like teenagers.

4. Multidisciplinary Care:

Medical Monitoring: Schedule regular check-ups to address physical health issues.

Psychological Intervention: Treatment for malformed thinking patterns might include cognitive-behavioral therapy (CBT).

Nutritional Support: Developing realistic and well-balanced meal plans in collaboration with nutritionists.

5. Family Engagement:

Family therapy: Involving family members in a patient's care may be very important, particularly for young people.

Resolving Fundamental Problems:

Developing Your Self-Esteem: Pay attention to your body image and self-esteem.

Coping Skills: Provide constructive coping strategies for handling stress and emotional difficulties.

6. Programs For Prevention:

School Programs: To encourage a good body image, implement awareness campaigns in schools.

Media literacy: Inform people about the power of the media and encourage them to question conventional notions of beauty.

To sum up, a thorough strategy for treating anorexia nervosa entails comprehending the condition's description, diagnostic standards, subtypes, and variations in addition to taking into account the many risk factors and etiological variables. In order to support a comprehensive recovery process, the simple solution approach places a strong emphasis on early intervention, interdisciplinary therapy, family participation, treating underlying psychological difficulties, and putting preventative measures into place.

CHAPTER THREE

Symptoms And Indications

Anorexia Nervosa Symptoms And Signs

1. Physical Expressions:

• Extreme Weight Loss: People who suffer from anorexia nervosa often lose a large amount of weight and keep it far below what is considered normal for their height and age.

• Physical Weakness and Fatigue: People who consume inadequate nourishment may become weak, tired, and lose general physical strength.

• Changes in Appearance: In an effort to keep the body warm, anorexia may cause a number of physical changes, including hair loss, brittle nails, and the growth of a thin covering of hair (lanugo) across the body.

• Menstrual irregularities: Anorexia in females may result in irregular menstrual periods amenorrhea or the lack of menstruation.

2. Behavioral Markers:

• Dietary limitations: Severe dietary limitations and the avoidance of certain food categories are often the result of an obsessive obsession with food, dieting, and calorie consumption.

• Excessive and obsessive Exercise: The need to burn calories and reduce weight sometimes leads to excessive and obsessive exercise.

• Social Withdrawal: People who suffer from anorexia may distance themselves from social situations, particularly those that include food, in order to avoid having to eat in front of others or answering inquiries about their eating patterns.

• Preoccupation with Body Image: Common behaviors linked to anorexia include constantly assessing one's appearance, expressing unhappiness with one's size or form, and having a skewed perspective of one's own body.

3. Signs of Emotion and Psychology:

• Extreme dread of Weight Gain: One of the main characteristics of anorexia nervosa is an intense dread of gaining weight or becoming "fat". Extreme actions to preserve low body weight are often motivated by this dread.

• Distorted Body Image: Despite evidence to the contrary, people who suffer from anorexia often have a mistaken perception of their body and consider themselves to be overweight.

• Mood Swings: The physical repercussions of malnutrition on the brain may contribute to emotional instability, irritability, and mood swings.

• Perfectionism: People with anorexia nervosa often have high levels of perfectionism, where they hold themselves to unreasonably high standards, especially when it comes to their physical appearance and weight.

Simplified Method Of Solving:

1. Early Intervention:

• Accurately identify the symptoms and indicators.

• Promote open communication and provide people with a safe venue to voice their worries without passing judgment.

2. Multidisciplinary Assistance:

• Assist a group of medical specialists, such as dietitians, psychiatrists, and mental health specialists, in addressing the psychological and medical components of anorexia.

3. Psychoeducation:

• Spread awareness of anorexia nervosa among people and their families, stressing the value of getting expert assistance and busting myths.

4. CBT, or cognitive-behavioral therapy:

• Use evidence-based treatment strategies, such as cognitive behavioral therapy (CBT), to address the erroneous beliefs and behaviors linked to anorexia.

5. Rehabilitation of Nutrition:

• Work together with nutritionists to create a customized, well-balanced diet plan, progressively reintroducing healthy eating to regain physical health.

6. Extended Assistance:

• Understand that getting well takes time and constant assistance. Put relapse prevention techniques into practice and create a strong network of allies.

7. Treat the underlying problems:

• Investigate and treat any underlying emotional, psychological, or environmental elements that may be influencing the onset of anorexia.

Recall that the path to anorexia nervosa recovery is intricate and needs a thorough, customized strategy. Involving medical experts and a network of support in the therapy process is crucial.

CHAPTER FOUR
Effects On The Body

A severe mental health condition known as anorexia nervosa is characterized by a person's warped body image and overwhelming dread of gaining weight, which drives them to follow restricted eating habits. Anorexia nervosa has a significant negative influence on physical health and may lead to a number of medical issues, long-term health issues, nutritional deficiencies, and organ damage.

1. Health Issues:

Cardiovascular Problems: Excessive calorie restriction may cause blood pressure and heart rate to drop. Irregular heartbeats, or arrhythmias, may occur, and the heart muscle may weaken. The risk of heart failure and abrupt cardiac arrest is raised by these cardiovascular alterations.

Electrolyte imbalance: Because anorexia nervosa often results in inadequate intake of vital minerals including potassium, sodium, and calcium, electrolyte imbalances are frequently caused by the disorder. This imbalance may have potentially fatal consequences by interfering with normal cardiac and muscular function.

Constipation, bloating, and stomach discomfort are just a few of the gastrointestinal problems that may result from chronic malnutrition. Long-term hunger may cause a disorder called gastroparesis, which impairs the stomach's ability to empty itself.

2. Long-Term Effects On Health:

Bone Health: Osteoporosis, a disorder marked by weakening and brittle bones, may be brought on by anorexia nervosa. Insufficient intake of certain nutrients, particularly calcium and vitamin D, raises the risk of fractures and skeletal abnormalities by decreasing bone density.

Reproductive Health: Amenorrhea, or the lack of menstruation, is a common menstrual cycle disturbance seen by women suffering from anorexia nervosa. Pregnancy risks and problems with conception might result from prolonged amenorrhea.

Cognitive Impairment: The brain is impacted by long-term starvation. Over time, memory loss, concentration problems, and cognitive deterioration are all possible in anorexics.

3. Inadequate Dietary Resources:

Vitamin and Mineral Deficiencies: Vitamin A, vitamin B12, iron, zinc, and other important vitamins and minerals are often deficient due to inadequate dietary consumption. These inadequacies have the potential to damage several body systems and be a factor in weariness, weakness, and immune system dysfunction.

Protein Deficiency: Weakness and muscular atrophy may result from consuming too little protein. Proteins are necessary for the upkeep and repair of tissues, and a lack of them may affect the body's structural integrity as a whole.

4. Organ Injury:

Long-term anorexia nervosa may result in multi-organ malfunction, which may harm the kidneys, liver, and other important organs. In order to get energy, the body starts to break down muscular tissue, which may further impair organ performance.

Immune System Compromised: People who are malnourished have weakened immune systems, which leaves them more vulnerable to infections and diseases. This heightened susceptibility may aggravate medical conditions and make recuperation more difficult.

In conclusion, anorexia nervosa presents serious risks to one's physical well-being because of its propensity for organ damage, long-term effects, and medical issues. Addressing these health concerns and fostering recovery need early intervention, which includes medical and dietary assistance. To manage anorexia nervosa and lessen its effects on physical health, a thorough and interdisciplinary strategy combining mental health specialists, medical doctors, and nutritionists is necessary.

CHAPTER FIVE
Aspects Psychological

Body image distortion is defined as a substantial misconception of one's own weight, size, or form. People who suffer from anorexia nervosa often have a skewed perception of their bodies, supposing themselves to be overweight even if they are underweight.

Factors That Contribute:

1. Cultural Influences: A skewed perception of one's physique might result from society's standards of thinness and attractiveness.

2. Media Influence: Unrealistic expectations may result from exposure to the media's idealized portrayals of bodies.

3. Peer Comparisons: Unrealistic beliefs may be fueled by constantly comparing oneself to others, particularly when it comes to physical appearance.

4. Biological Factors: According to some studies, body image distortion may be inherited.

Method Of Treatment:

1. Cognitive-Behavioral Therapy (CBT): Body image-related distortions in thought processes are often addressed with CBT. It supports people in questioning and altering harmful mental patterns.

2. Mirror Exposure Therapy: This modifies perceptions by progressively increasing the amount of time spent gazing at oneself in a mirror.

3. Acceptance and Commitment Therapy (ACT): This method focuses on making good behaviors a commitment while acknowledging the thoughts and emotions related to body image distortion.

Control And Perfectionism:

Definition: Those suffering from anorexia nervosa often exhibit perfectionism and a desire for control. Seeking a desired body weight turns into a means of taking charge of one's life.

Factors That Contribute:

1. Psychological Factors: The need to live up to high expectations and win others over is a common source of perfectionism.

2. Environmental Factors: Restricting food intake may be an effort to manage stress or erratic circumstances in life.

3. Personality qualities that tend to tilt toward perfectionism and a desire for control are common among anorexics.

Method Of Treatment:

1. Dialectical Behavior Therapy (DBT): DBT may assist people in creating more healthy coping strategies for managing their emotions and stress.

2. Nutritional counseling: Learning about a balanced diet might assist people in letting go of strict dietary restrictions.

3. Mindfulness Practices: Managing the need for perfection may be aided by methods such as mindfulness meditation.

Typical Co-occurring Conditions:

1. Depression: Feelings of worthlessness and depression are common side effects of anorexia nervosa.

2. Anxiety Disorders: Anorexia may coexist with obsessive-compulsive disorder, social anxiety, or generalized anxiety.

3.   Substance Abuse: As a coping mechanism for mental anguish, people with anorexia may abuse substances.

4.   Personality Disorders: Anorexia may coexist with borderline personality disorder or other personality disorders.

Method Of Treatment:

1.   Integrated Treatment Plans: For a full recovery, treating co-occurring illnesses and anorexia at the same time is essential.

2.   Medication: To treat the symptoms of co-occurring disorders, doctors may sometimes prescribe medication.

3.   In supportive psychotherapy, forming a therapeutic relationship is crucial to addressing many concerns at once.

It's critical to comprehend how perfectionism, body image distortion, and comorbidity with other mental health conditions interact in order to develop treatment plans that work for anorexics. Comprehensive treatment often requires a multidisciplinary approach combining medical doctors, dietitians, and mental health specialists.

CHAPTER SIX
Social Factors

In this section, we'll examine the sociocultural elements that contribute to the onset and maintenance of anorexia nervosa, with a particular emphasis on the role played by the media and culture, social pressures and expectations, stigma, and misunderstandings.

Cultural And Media Factors:

1. Ideals of Body Image:

The media, which includes social media, television, and publications, often promotes unattainable body standards. The abundance of photos with abnormally slim models might cause people to internalize these standards and develop a skewed view of their own bodies.

2. Influence of Celebrities:

Public personalities and celebrities often set the bar for success and attractiveness. Constant exposure to pictures of slender, apparently perfect celebrities may perpetuate unattainable body ideals and foster a society that prioritizes thinness above health.

3. Marketing and Promotion:

Advertising usually equates pleasure, success, and attractiveness with being skinny. Images that support a certain body image are often used in the marketing of goods and services, promoting the notion that obtaining or maintaining such a physique is necessary for both social approval and personal pleasure.

Social Expectations And Pressures:

1. Influence from peers:

One important component is the desire to blend in and be accepted by peers. Particularly adolescents and young adults are susceptible to social pressure, which may lead them to adopt restrictive eating habits in an effort to fit in with society's standards.

2. Family Relationships:

Anorexia nervosa may arise as a result of family dynamics and relationships. An individual's susceptibility to eating disorders may be worsened by unfulfilled expectations from family members, unhealthy communication styles, or an emphasis on outward appearance rather than general well-being.

3. Stress in Education and the Workplace:

Excessive stress brought on by success in school or the workplace may either cause or worsen anorexia nervosa. Anxiety to succeed and live up to social norms about achievement may result in unhealthy coping strategies, such as obsessive dieting.

Stereotypes And Stigma:

1. Misperceptions about the Disorder:

Stigma is exacerbated by common beliefs about anorexia nervosa. The idea that it's just a matter of lifestyle or a need for attention might impede empathy and the provision of necessary help. It's a common misconception that those who suffer from anorexia nervosa may easily "snap out of it."

2.   Stigmatization of Culture:

Eating disorders and other mental health conditions may be stigmatized in certain societies. This societal stigma may discourage people from asking for assistance, which may result in insufficient or delayed care.

3.   Sensationalism and Media Representation:

Eating disorders are sensationalized by the media a lot, which results in damaging and false representations. This may reinforce negative preconceptions and further isolate those who are dealing with anorexia nervosa.

In conclusion, treating anorexia nervosa necessitates a multifaceted strategy that takes into account and confronts cultural factors. This includes encouraging positive peer and family situations, encouraging realistic body portrayals in the media, and using education and awareness efforts to fight stigma. Establishing a culture that prioritizes individual well-being, diversity, and mental health above damaging cultural conventions is crucial.

CHAPTER SEVEN
Methods of Therapy

1. Medical Procedures:

Bedding in:

Hospitalization may be necessary for severe instances of anorexia nervosa in order to treat serious health issues such as organ failure, electrolyte imbalances, and malnourishment. This entails dietary therapy, medical supervision, and often the intravenous delivery of nutrients.

Drugs:

Medications may be used to treat co-occurring illnesses and manage symptoms. Mood disorders may be treated with antidepressants, such as selective serotonin reuptake inhibitors (SSRIs). If there are notable symptoms of anxiety or psychosis, antipsychotics or anti-anxiety drugs may be prescribed.

Dietary Advice:

Throughout the medical intervention process, registered dietitians are essential because they develop customized meal plans, inform patients about their nutritional requirements, and help them develop a positive connection with food.

2. Counseling And Psychotherapy:

CBT, or cognitive-behavioral therapy:

One of the most popular treatment modalities for anorexia nervosa is cognitive behavioral therapy. It assists people in recognizing and altering skewed mentalities and actions around food, weight, and body image. When it comes to treating the underlying psychological issues that are causing the condition, CBT works well.

Treatment for Dialectical Behavior (DBT):

DBT focuses on developing skills related to mindfulness, distress tolerance, emotion regulation, and interpersonal efficacy. Those with anorexia nervosa who have emotional dysregulation may benefit most from it.

Psychotherapy that is interpersonal (IPT):

IPT focuses on interpersonal problems and relationships, assisting people with anorexia nervosa in examining and resolving social and interpersonal challenges that could be involved in the onset or maintenance of the illness.

3. Family-Centered Care:

The Maudsley Method:

The family is actively involved in the therapy process using this evidence-based approach. Refeeding their kid and gradually returning control to the person as they make progress toward recovery are important roles that parents play.

Family Counseling:

The goals of family therapy are to enhance family system communication and settle disputes. It recognizes the role that family relations have in the onset and upkeep of anorexia nervosa.

4. Complementary And Holistic Therapies:

Expressive arts and therapy:

Dance, music, or art therapy may be helpful in offering different avenues for self-expression and exploration. These techniques may assist people in exploring and expressing their feelings nonverbally.

Yoga and Intentionality:

Mind-body techniques, like yoga and mindfulness, may help people feel more connected to their bodies, become more self-aware, and experience less anxiety.

Both massage and acupuncture:

Complementary treatments, like massage or acupuncture, may help some people relax and manage their stress. These may be included in a more comprehensive wellness plan, even if they shouldn't take the place of evidence-based therapies.

To summarize, an integrated treatment strategy for anorexia nervosa often combines medical, psychological, and holistic approaches customized to meet the unique requirements of the patient. A thorough and successful treatment strategy must take into account the disorder's complexity and address both the physical and psychological components.

CHAPTER EIGHT
Healing And Preventing Relapses

An extreme fear of gaining weight is the hallmark of anorexia nervosa, a complicated mental health illness that causes severe dietary restrictions and other maladaptive behaviors.

Although the road to rehabilitation is difficult, it is necessary to regain both mental and physical well-being. In order to fully recover from an illness, both its psychological and physical components must be addressed, with an emphasis on long-term well-being.

Phases Of Rehab:

1. Recognition and Acceptance:

• Admitting that there is a problem and that assistance is required is the first step.

• Helping people understand how their actions affect their relationships and overall health.

2. Medical Grounding:

• Taking care of any urgent medical issues, such as electrolyte imbalances, malnourishment, and other medical issues.

• Working together with healthcare providers to create a customized treatment strategy.

3. Rehabilitation of Nutrition:

• Assisting nutritionists in creating a sustainable and well-balanced food plan.

• Spreading knowledge about healthy eating and ending the loop of restricted eating habits.

4. Intervention for Therapy:

• Seeking treatment for erroneous beliefs and actions via psychotherapy, such as dialectical behavior therapy (DBT) or cognitive-behavioral therapy (CBT).

• Looking at underlying problems, such as self-esteem, perfectionism, and body image difficulties.

5. Developing Resilience:

• Dispensing practical coping skills for handling stress, worry, and emotional upset.

• Endorsing more healthful means of expressing feelings and handling difficult circumstances.

6. Planning for Relapse Prevention:

• Creating a comprehensive strategy to avoid relapses in conjunction with therapists and support systems.

• Recognizing warning indicators and putting plans in place to act before a relapse happens.

Obstacles And Relapse Precursors:

1. Issues with Body Image:

• Perturbed body image continues to be a major obstacle. It takes ongoing therapeutic interventions to modify and normalize views.

2. Social Coercion:

Relapse may be influenced by cultural norms and societal expectations. It is essential to develop resilience against outside forces.

3. Perfectiveness:

• Constant attention is needed to address the perfectionistic inclinations that often accompany anorexia. It is crucial to promote a more adaptable way of thinking.

4. Triggers for Emotions:

• It is essential to recognize and control emotional triggers. Refinement of coping mechanisms is necessary to handle changing emotional difficulties.

5. Absence of Assistance:

Isolation may result from inadequate support systems. It is essential to strengthen ties with family, friends, and support networks.

Techniques For Long-Term Recuperation:

1. Extended Therapeutic Interaction:

• Encouraging patients to continue seeing a therapist even after they have made some progress.

• Routine check-ins with mental health specialists might assist in addressing new problems.

2. Knowledge and Consciousness:

• Encouraging continued education on mental health, nutrition, and the long-term effects of eating disorders.

• Increasing knowledge of one's own triggers and useful coping techniques.

3. Being Aware and Being Kind to Oneself:

• Using self-compassion and mindfulness exercises to promote a better connection with oneself on a daily basis.

4. Encouragement Setting:

• Fostering a welcoming atmosphere that promotes candid discussion of setbacks and victories.

• Including friends and family in the healing process.

5. A Holistic Perspective on Health:

• Placing emphasis on a comprehensive view of health that takes emotional, mental, and physical well-being into account.

• Including practices that enhance general well-being, such as consistent exercise, enough sleep, and stress reduction.

6. Honoring Significant Occasions:

• Highlighting and applauding individual accomplishments, regardless of size, to support development and inspiration.

To sum up, the process of recovering from anorexia nervosa is complex, requiring the implementation of sustainable techniques, addressing specific obstacles, and going through many phases. The secret is to take a thorough, customized strategy that prioritizes long-term well-being while taking into account the disorder's complex nature. To sustain long-term recovery and avoid relapse, family, friends, and medical professionals must provide unwavering support.

CHAPTER NINE
Assistive Systems

The Value Of A Helpful Environment:

1. Emotional Balance:

• A complex interaction of psychological, emotional, and social elements often results in anorexia nervosa. Emotional stability may be greatly enhanced by a supportive atmosphere that creates a feeling of safety and comprehension.

2. Cutting Down on Isolation

• People who are anorexic may withdraw from others out of fear or embarrassment. A support network may help combat this loneliness by offering company and a judgment-free environment conducive to candid conversation.

3. Inspiration and Encouragement:

• Encouragement and motivation are essential for overcoming anorexia. Positive reinforcement from a supportive atmosphere might help people remain motivated throughout the difficult recovery process.

4. Developing Self-Belief:

• Low self-esteem and a distorted body image are common symptoms of anorexia nervosa. Sustained rehabilitation requires the development of confidence and self-worth, both of which may be greatly aided by a supportive atmosphere.

Family And Friends' Roles:

1. Comprehending and Feeling:

• Friends and family are essential in helping people with anorexia appreciate the difficulties they experience. Building empathy lessens stigma and aids in the creation of a safe environment for candid conversation.

2. Cooperative Care:

• Treatment is more successful when friends and family are involved. They may actively engage in educational initiatives, family counseling, and therapy sessions, supporting a rehabilitation strategy that is all-encompassing.

3. Observation and Assistance:

• Family members may help with medication compliance, food habit monitoring, and emotional support during trying times. Their participation fosters an atmosphere that is responsible and organized.

4. Learning:

• Friends and family may educate themselves on the signs and symptoms of anorexia nervosa as well as the process of recovery. This lowers the possibility of inadvertent triggers and empowers them to provide knowledgeable help.

Resources In The Community And Advocacy:

1. Expert Assistance:

• It is essential to have access to mental health specialists, such as therapists, nutritionists, and support groups. Professional assistance should be easily and affordably available via community resources.

2. Advocacy Organizations:

• A large portion of the community's assistance comes from groups that promote eating disorder prevention and mental health awareness. These organizations are able to plan events, lead awareness campaigns, and provide resources for people and their support systems.

3. Programs for Education:

• Community-based educational initiatives may lessen stigma, encourage early intervention, and debunk misconceptions about anorexia nervosa. Community centers, businesses, and schools all provide excellent locations for these kinds of initiatives.

4. Crisis Intervention Services:

• Medical crises may result from anorexia nervosa. Crisis intervention services should be part of the community's resources to guarantee prompt aid in moments of extreme distress.

In summary, the development of a strong support network has to be the first priority in any streamlined strategy for treating anorexia nervosa. In order to establish a complete network for people on the road to recovery, it is necessary to cultivate a supportive atmosphere, acknowledge the critical role that friends and family play, and make use of community resources and advocacy.

Conclusion

In summary, treating anorexia nervosa requires a thorough and multifaceted strategy that extends beyond conventional medical measures. It is important to comprehend the intricacies of this mental health condition in order to devise efficacious approaches for intervention, support, and prevention. The significance of a streamlined solution strategy that prioritizes raising awareness and compassion should be emphasized in the conclusion.

Summary Of Main Ideas:

Recognizing that anorexia nervosa is a significant mental health problem marked by extreme dietary restriction, a distorted body image, and an acute fear of gaining weight is the first step toward understanding the condition. It's critical to debunk popular myths and misunderstandings about anorexia in order to advance truthful knowledge.

Multifaceted Nature: Anorexia nervosa is a complicated illness that is influenced by social, psychological, and biological aspects. Achieving sustained recovery requires a comprehensive approach to therapy that takes these different aspects into account.

Early Intervention: Improving the prognosis for those suffering from anorexia nervosa requires early identification and intervention. Further decline in both physical and psychological functioning may be avoided by recognizing warning indicators and offering assistance in the early stages of the illness.

Holistic therapy Strategy: A holistic therapy strategy should address the underlying psychological difficulties, such as distorted body image, poor self-esteem, and perfectionism, rather than only concentrating on weight restoration. Anorexia nervosa has been effectively treated using therapeutic techniques including cognitive-behavioral therapy (CBT) and family-based treatment (FBT).

Nutritional Rehabilitation: A vital component of recovery, nutritional rehabilitation is just as important as psychological therapy. In order to restore physical health, it is essential to collaborate with licensed dietitians and nutritionists to create a customized, balanced eating plan.

Peer and Family Support: Considering the value of social support, a person's rehabilitation may be facilitated by including family members and peers in the therapeutic process. Overcoming the obstacles posed by anorexia nervosa requires establishing a supportive atmosphere that encourages comprehension and empathy.

Education and knowledge: Reducing stigma and promoting early intervention for anorexia nervosa needs to raise public knowledge of the condition. Educational initiatives in businesses, communities, and schools may help debunk stereotypes, promote empathy, and make the environment more accepting of those who are dealing with the illness.

The Way Ahead: Promoting Consciousness And Empathy

In the future, cultivating compassion and understanding at the individual and social levels should be the main priorities. This includes:

Enacting educational initiatives in schools and communities to raise awareness of the warning signs, symptoms, and aftereffects of anorexia nervosa is known as "promoting education." As a result, society may become more knowledgeable and kind.

Reducing Stigma: It's critical to address the stigma attached to anorexia nervosa in order to empower people to ask for assistance without worrying about being judged. Fostering candid dialogue and comprehension may help create a more encouraging atmosphere.

Promoting Compassionate Language: It is crucial to promote the use of nonjudgmental, compassionate language while talking about anorexia nervosa.

Supporting study: To further our knowledge of anorexia nervosa and provide more potent therapies, more study is required on the disorder's causes and treatments. Research activities that get support may help the field develop.

To sum up, a comprehensive treatment strategy, early intervention techniques, acceptance of the disorder's complexity, and cultivation of compassion and awareness are all components of a simple solution approach to anorexia nervosa. Together, people, communities, and healthcare systems can address these crucial issues and provide a more understanding and supportive environment for those who suffer from anorexia nervosa.

THE END